Healthy Living & Nutrition Simplified

By: Jerry Reeves

Second Edition

Table of Contents

Introduction

Following a nutritional diet is a lifestyle change. It contributes to a healthier you and can improve your general well being. *Healthy Living and Nutrition Simplified* will provide you with a better understanding of how to achieve optimum health through a nutritional diet.

The aim of this book is to:

- Improve your understanding of nutrition by providing you with information about the different food groups and how they benefit your health.
- Look at various physical activities and how they can contribute to your health.
- Set you up for the future by giving you a plan of action which, when correctly followed, will create a way of living that is easy to follow and maintain.
- Recognize foods that negatively affect your health and provide you with ways to eradicate them from your diet.

The goal is to give you a better understanding about maintaining optimum health, as well as learning how to avoid various diet-related diseases like heart disease, diabetes, obesity etc. You will also find out how following a nutritional diet can have a positive impact on your mind and body, learning how to achieve a better physical and mental state.

Hopefully, as you read through the book you will discover why crash and fad diets never work. You will also learn about the benefits of drinking water for cleansing and purification. As well as looking at nutrition, this book will also provide you with information about exercising and various physical activities that will not only support your weight loss, but will also improve your stamina.

Healthy Living and Nutrition Simplified adopts a clear approach and will provide you with a realistic set of goals that you can achieve to adapt your lifestyle and your diet, improving your work, home life and overall wellbeing.

Chapter 1: Nutrition And Healthy Living

Healthy Heart

A healthy lifestyle is extremely important in maintaining a healthy heart, with a lot of heart disease being a direct result of a bad diet. The most common types of heart disease are related to high blood pressure. High blood pressure occurs when the blood flow in your arteries are too strong, producing small cracks. When they are repaired it leads to the artery walls thickening and consequently results in problems with blood flow along with a risk of blockages and clotting. Once blood flow has reduced, there is less of a supply to your vital organs, which results in tissue death. High blood pressure is often the cause of heart attacks, heart failure, strokes and even kidney failure. The great news is that high blood pressure can be managed with a healthy diet and lifestyle.

Below is a list of a healthy-living plan to improve and maintain a healthy heart:

- Reduce your intake of salt/sodium.
- Exercise regularly and maintain a healthy weight.
- Reduce and limit your intake of alcohol and ideally stop smoking.
- Manage stress levels.

A diet to ensure a healthy heart should include:

- A minimum of 4 ½ cups of fruit and veg daily.

- A 3 ½ ounce serving of fish each week.
- No more than 1,500 mg of sodium daily.
- Less than 400 calories of sugary drinks each week.
- A minimum of 4 services of legumes, nuts and seeds each week.
- A maximum of 2 servings of processed meat each week.

Reducing your risk of diseases

Unfortunately, cancer is becoming an increasingly common occurrence in our modern society. A lot of research has been done that examines how diet relates to the development of certain cancers. Studies actually show that increasing your consumption of fruit, vegetables and grains can actually restrict the growth of cancer within various parts of the body including lung, prostate and colon. Below is a list of nutrients that professionals believe will reduce the risk of cancer:

Antioxidants

Antioxidants are a substance that prevents oxidative damage. They defend the body against free radicals – the result of a natural body process – that can damage healthy cells, changing the structure of DNA resulting in tumorous growths. Antioxidants can be found in:

- Vitamin C, which is in green peppers, oranges, strawberries (raw), red peppers (raw), papaya and broccoli.
- Pro vitamin A which is in cabbage, green spinach, carrots, collards, squash and sweet potatoes. .
- Vitamin E, which is in sunflower oil/seeds, hazelnuts, almonds, peanuts and wheat bread.

Omega-3 fatty acids

Omega-3 fatty acids can be found in foods such as: kidney beans, flaxseed oil, soybeans and seafood – cold-water fish in particular.

Phytochemicals

Phytochemicals is a chemical compound that is found naturally in plants. It can be found in fruit and vegetables (broccoli, berries, apricots, onions, cabbage and so on), beans, whole grain cereals/grains and even wine. Phytochemicals have different benefits depending on the type of food that they are found in, from acting as an antioxidant to preventing carcinogens from developing.

Healthy Mind

Research suggests that there is a strong link between nutrition and mental health, with a good diet having a positive impact. An innutritious diet is said to have a damaging effect on mental health with issues such as Alzheimer's, Attention Deficit Hyperactivity Disorder, Schizophrenia and depression – and their prevention, management and development.

There have been various studies carried out that suggest eating healthily can have a positive impact on mental health. By sticking to a balanced diet - with the right amount of essential fats, complex carbohydrates, vitamins, minerals and water – you can be assured that your mind and wellbeing will remain as healthy as possible.

Tryptophan, an amino acid, is said to improve your mood. It naturally occurs in protein and therefore, you should aim to have a source of protein with each meal. Foods that are high in protein include meat, eggs, milk, fish, nuts, cheese, beans and even some meat substitutes.

As well as eating healthily to maintain a healthy mind, mental exercises are also beneficial and there are many different ways to do this. Ideally, you should try and exercise your brain daily whether that is through doing crosswords, playing scrabble or even choosing not to use a calculator. There are also various games that are specifically designed to exercise the brain.

Reading is also very important in keeping the brain active. It does not have to be anything comprehensive, a newspaper will do. You could also take up a new hobby, it is an easy way to maintain a healthy mind; doing something you like is enjoyable and demands a certain level of concentration.

Feel Better, Live Longer

Sometimes you may find that even after a good night's sleep you are still dozing off during the day, and this can be down to your diet. What you choose to eat has a significant impact on your level of energy, with some foods sapping your levels and others giving you that needed boost. Eating a balanced and healthy diet, with a good amount of nutrients and keeping yourself hydrated, you will find that you have a lot more energy.

A common misconception with a healthy eating plan is that you need to eat a lot less, with some choosing to skip meals. However, this can have a negative impact on your energy as it can cause your blood sugar levels to fluctuate, which can leave you feeling extremely lethargic. Ideally, you should be eating a minimum of three meals a day, although four to six meals spread throughout the day are even better for energy maintenance. Ensuring you have enough protein in your diet will also increase your levels of energy, as it stabilizes your blood glucose levels, especially after consuming a lot of carbohydrates.

Additionally, having an adequate level of iron in your body is essential in boosting your energy, with one of the first symptoms of an iron deficiency being severe fatigue. Iron naturally occurs in some food including fortified cereals, dried beans, fruits, nuts, seeds, red meat and fish. As our bodies find it difficult to absorb iron, eating foods rich in vitamin C should support that process.

The University of Otago did a study on the relationship between fruit and vegetables and our emotions. Unsurprisingly, they found that young people who ate the most fruit and vegetables, tended to feel calmer, energetic and generally a lot happier.

The study consisted of 281 young people, with an average age of 20, keeping an online food diary for 21 days. They were required to write down what they had eaten based on five questions that they were given, as well as having to rate their emotions by using nine adjectives for positive feelings and nine for negative. One of the questions they were given was to answer how many servings of fresh fruit and vegetables they had eaten - not counting juices and dried fruit. Additionally, they were questioned about a few unhealthy food choices including cookies, muffins and potato chips.

The study resulted in some interesting findings. There was a significant link between diet and the participants' emotions, with the intake of fruit and vegetables seemingly having a positive effect on their mood – a lot happier, calmer and more energetic than they usually feel.

From this investigation, the researchers believe that to feel these positive effects from fruit and vegetables, people would need to consume around seven to eight portions daily. The type of portion size you would need is roughly half a cup, or a handful. Although, the study showed a hopeful connection between a healthy diet and a positive mood, a more extensive study is required to demonstrate the real benefits.

Inevitably, eating healthy foods supports your immune system and as a result will increase your life span. It is important to eat a nutritionally balanced diet to avoid becoming malnourished as that can lead to free radicals and oxidative damage. As part of a healthy diet, your intake of glycolysis naturally decreases while lipid metabolism raises, and glycolysis reduction has been said to add years to your life.

A healthy eating plan can also improve your life span by reducing the risk of diseases associated with a bad diet including but not limited to cancer, a stroke, heart disease and diabetes. By simply sticking to a natural and nutritional diet and regularly exercising, you can lower your risk of developing such diseases. Although, a healthy diet can be associated with an increased life span, there are also other factors involved including good medical care, excellent hygiene and overall clean living. Regular exercise is also a must. Statistically, those living a sedentary life tend to have a lower life expectancy.

Sense of Achievement
Having a nutritionally balanced diet along with an adequate amount of physical activity, you will find that your life improves dramatically. Not only will you feel good, you will have the satisfaction of knowing that your mind and body are strong, you have more energy and feel happier all round.

Look Better, Feel Great
Essentially, the skin is the largest organ and so it needs to be treated accordingly. Just like other organs in the body, the skin responds similarly to a healthy diet, regular exercise and a good night's sleep. To achieve a great complexion it is unnecessary to spend a fortune on products, as just adapting your lifestyle slightly is extremely effective.

Here are some great changes that you can make to your diet:
Fish: As well as being great for your health, fish is also great for complexion, which is why it is an essential component in the Mediterranean Diet. Most types of fish will work, but oysters and oily fish like salmon are the most effective.

Zinc: Zinc is good for the skin, and works especially well at fighting acne. It also supports cell production and the regeneration of skin, leaving it looking radiant. Zinc occurs naturally in citrus fruits, but supplements are more effective.

Vitamin C: Vitamin C is great for the complexion, which is why it is an ingredient in so many beauty products. It supports the product of collagen in the body – a protein that is part of the basic skin structure and it is the breakdown of collagen, which leaves you skin looking saggy. By eating more foods that are rich in vitamin C – grapefruits, oranges, acerola cherries and tomatoes – tighten the skin and reduce the appearance of wrinkles. Orange and red vegetables are good to eat as they are packed with beta-carotene, which are body converts to vitamin A, acting as an antioxidant.

Vitamin A: Vitamin A aids the skin in the regeneration of cells, minimizing dryness and leaving your skin looking young and radiant. Green and leafy foods, like spinach, will provide you with an adequate amount of Vitamin A, Mangoes are also good.

Vitamin E: Vitamin E is good at combating the appearance of ageing. The vitamin fights free radicals associated with skin ageing – protecting against sun damage. It also supports the skin in retaining moisture, diminishing dryness and leaves it looking fresh.

Vitamin B: Vitamin B biotin occurs in whole grains such as wheat. It supports the cells with processing fats; without biotin your skin can appear dry and flakey.

Having the right nutrients in your body is extremely beneficial for your skin and with fresh looking skin you will feel confident. By improving your physical appearance as well as your skin the effects will double leaving you feeling amazing all round. You can do this by adopting a healthy and nutritional diet and taking part in regular exercise; this way your skin will look great and your physical appearance.

If your diet consists of regularly eating junk food and fast food, it will eventually lead to a significant weight gain, while wreaking havoc on your skin. This happens because these types of foods are laden with saturated fats, extremely greasy and offer no nutritional benefits. Our bodies are not built to process these foods therefore leaving us with a string of problems. In contrast, eating fresh fruit and vegetables and other non-processed foods will not increase your weight, but will give you all the nutrients that will leave you looking and feeling great.

There are many different foods that you can eat that are good for your skin and body including: apricots, carrots, vegetables, spinach, blueberries, tomatoes, peas, beans, lentils, nuts and fish. Foods that you want to avoid are those that contain a large amount of fat, sugar and salt, these are foods that can aggravate skin that already suffers some form of irritation. As well as leaving you looking better, you will also feel a lot better as your immune system will get that added boost. Your energy will also improve.

If you find it difficult to adopt these changes, you may want to find someone close to you to emulate. Brown University's Student Health Services carried out some research on the development of a practical body image. They found that being around someone you know that has a good relationship with food, exercise and their general wellbeing can you do wonders.

Chapter 2: Why Changing Your Lifestyle Works and Crash Dieting Doesn't

In our modern society, obesity is becoming increasingly common and widespread. Many people still have this preconceived idea that overnight solutions and quick fixes truly work. However, in reality they never do – the weight will soon pile back on - and can actually have an extremely bad effect on your health. Crash diets are always promoted as a quick way to lose weight, which is why so many dieters try it. In truth, the rapid weight loss – which usually only occurs in the first week – is a result of the body going into shock and then starvation mode and the weight loss is in fact water and glycogen. Although this may give you the quick fix you hoped for, it is also putting your health at risk from a range of problems including malnourishment and more serious issues like osteoporosis and damage to your vital organs.

These types of diet can also affect your mood significantly from minor irritation to severe fatigue and sometimes even depression simply because your body is not getting enough nutrients. Additionally, by being malnourished, your body will naturally crave food, as it needs vitamins and minerals to function. Crash diets generally have a low success rate because the weight goes back on as soon as it comes off. As most of these diets involve restricting what you eat, the body goes into starvation mode, which lowers your metabolism meaning you do not burn as much calories. Once you have finished the program and your diet returns to normal, the weight will be put back on even quicker.

Very few of us can say that we follow a totally healthy diet, with most of us consuming more calories than we need which is why obesity is becoming so widespread, along with a range of other weight-related health issues. As crash diets are so unsuccessful and risky, healthy eating and regular exercise is a much better approach to weight loss. Increasing your physical activity will increase the amount of calories you burn, setting the metabolic rate higher.

It may be difficult when you are first starting out, especially as you are conscious that it is a long-term change, rather than a two-week stint. Patience is essential when you begin to feel like this as you will quickly start to reap the benefits, from more energy to looking trimmer. Also, once the body becomes familiarized with your diet change, it will no longer crave for food, making the whole process a lot easier.

Chapter 3: Set Realistic Goals

Changing your lifestyle does take time, as it requires a certain amount of effort and planning. You should expect some difficulty, as the changes you will make will be habits that have slowly become engrained into your system throughout the years. You should take one step at a time and slowly adjust to new changes, as it will take a while to adapt. Exercise should also be approached in a similar way, slowly introduce yourself to physical activities, even if you begin with 20 minutes a week. What you shouldn't do is expect any overnight changes, weight takes longer to come off than be put on, be prepared to lose around two pounds per week – less is fine but any more than three pounds is an unhealthy rate.

Some days will be harder than others and you may find that you have momentary lapses, but do not let this discourage you as it is part of changing your eating habits, and happens to everyone. What you should do is acknowledge that you have strayed slightly and make a quick return to your eating plan. Do not wait until the next day to restart your diet, do it immediately, otherwise you may find 'tomorrow' turning into weeks.

An important component to weight loss is to be realistic, as setting unattainable goals, will leave you feeling disappointed and discouraged. Before you begin your diet, set a goal that you hope to achieve by a certain frame of time. This will make the process a lot easier and when you reach your goals, you will feel spurred on to achieve more, keeping you feeling motivated.

Below are some examples of goals:

Next week I am going to…
- Change to semi-skimmed milk.
- Go for a low-fat spread.
- Not skip breakfast.
- Only snack on nuts and fruit.
- Use stairs whenever I can.
- Lose 2lbs.

Chapter 4: Keeping Track

On average, dieters who monitor all aspects of their progress - food, activities and weight loss – tend to lose more weight than those who don't. What use is there in setting goals if you do not keep track of them?

By tracking your goals, you will know whether you manage to reach them or not, and what progress you are actually making. What is great about this is when you reach your goal you can give yourself a small treat, whether that is a muffin or a new blouse. It is also a way of knowing whether your goals are realistic or even too easy, you may even find yourself wanting more of a challenge.

Keeping a food and activity diary

Keeping track of what you eat and how much activity you do each day is extremely important. By writing down what you eat and drink, you can keep track on exactly what you are consuming. It is a way of monitoring eating habits, and can sometimes be quite an eye opener. You may be shocked by how much you eat or how little, it will also give you an idea of why you manage to lose or not lose weight that week. Similarly, monitoring your physical activity will help in building up the bigger picture.

To make your food and activity diary more effective, you should include a section for emotions, this way you can look at how you were feeling and what you were thinking. It will give you an insight into how you feel and what you eat. Often, there are certain emotional triggers that can set you off on a path of comfort eating. Seeing it written down and identifying the relationships between food and emotion will help you break the pattern.

Chapter 5: Portion Control

As part of a healthy eating plan you need to thinking about portion sizes and what you are eating. As well as eating a healthy variety of foods, you will want to control how much you are eating so that you do not overeat but just consume an adequate amount. A portion or serving size is the amount you eat for a meal, whether at home or in a restaurant. The amount you are required to eat daily is dependent on various factors including how old you are, what gender, your weight and level of activity. For instance, if a woman is 150 lbs. and exercises a lot, she will probably need to consume more calories than a woman who is a similar size but only walks for 20 minutes a week. There is no rule of how many calories one needs to consume or how much exercise is needed as it really does vary from person to person.

To ensure that you are not overeating, a handy trick is to always make sure that your food is served on a plate, rather than from a bag or a box. It can also be useful to serve your food on smaller dishes to trick your mind into thinking you are eating more than you actually are.

With whatever food you eat, the packaging will often tell you the nutritional information per serving. It is important that you follow the portions carefully; measuring out if that is what is needed. This way you know the nutritional value of whatever you are eating and can prevent yourself from consuming too much. Snacks should be approached in the same way. If you buy a large bag or box, you should divide them into single-serve portion sizes to ensure that you do not get carried away.

You should also avoid consuming your meal in front of the television or during other activities that require your attention. When you are eating a meal, you should focus on the task at hand, taking time to eat slowly, chewing properly and just really enjoying the taste and smell of your meal. Eating slowly will relay to your brain that your stomach is full, which can take nearly 20 minutes.

Chapter 6: The Importance of Drinking Water

Our body is around 70% water, making it a vital part of our being. Ensuring that you drink enough water each day is extremely beneficial for your health and wellbeing, as hydrating your body, will improve its efficiency, increase stamina and even fight against ageing.

Keeping your body hydrated is essential at preventing illness as it flushes your system, which also leaves your skin fresher and healthier. If exercise is a major part of your life, then it is even more important that you drink an adequate amount of water as psychical activity often leads to dehydration. To remain healthy, you need to drink at least four pints of water each day and while plain water is encouraged you could add a twist such as lemon or whatever you desire. Avoid drinks that dehydrate the body like coffee, tea and soda – generally drinks that have a high content of caffeine.

Below are some health benefits of drinking water:

Calorie control
Drinking water has been part of dieting for many years. This is because it is good for filling you up, but does not contain calories unlike other drinks. This way, you do not waste your calories on beverages and can use them on food instead.

Good skin
As well as being great for your health, water is also good for the skin. Although it cannot remove existing wrinkles, it can hydrate the skin making it look less dry and wrinkly.

Energizes muscles
It is said that Muscles tend to perform better when they are properly hydrated; this is because loss of fluid can lead to muscle fatigue.

Supports Kidneys
Your kidneys need water in order to do their job effectively. Water helps them cleanse your body, removing toxins that could are potentially harmful, but without the right amount of fluids it becomes more difficult.

Chapter 7: Why You Shouldn't Avoid All Fats?

There is a common misbelief amongst many nutritionists and dietitians that if you want to lose weight and achieve a healthy body, then you should avoid all types of fact. However, it is not that you should avoid fats all together, but really the type of fat you eat and how much you eat it. Consuming fat that is classed as bad for you will increase your risk of high cholesterol and various other types of health issues. Whereas if you consume good fats such as Omega-3, it can actually have a positive effect on your health as they are extremely good for your heart.

There has been a significant rise of low-fat foods being offered as an alternative to your favorite regulars, from low-fat yoghurt to light potato chips. While these guilt-free options are readily available, the level of obesity is still on the rise. Dieters are being given the wrong advice in avoiding fat completely, or sticking to low fat options. It is only unhealthy fats that are bad for your health, they are what cause diet-related conditions such as blocked arteries, obesity etc. Eating good fats – polyunsaturated, monounsaturated and omega-3s- actually have a good effect on your health. They help regulate your mood, improve your mental performance, give you energy and help with weight maintenance.

You should never eradicate fat out of your diet, but learn how to make healthy decisions in swapping them with good fats. As it is difficult to understand the various types of fats, it is important to have a clear break down. There are four significant types of fats: polyunsaturated, monounsaturated, saturated and trans-fat. Polyunsaturated and monounsaturated fats are good for your health, heart and cholesterol.

Polyunsaturated fats can be found in:
- Soybean oil, Corn oil and Safflower oil
- Walnuts
- Sunflower, sesame, and pumpkin seeds
- Flaxseed
- Fatty fish (salmon, tuna, mackerel, herring, trout, sardines)

Monounsaturated Fats are found in:
- Olive oil
- Canola oil
- Sunflower oil
- Peanut oil
- Sesame oil
- Avocados
- Olives
- Nuts (almonds, peanuts, macadamia nuts, hazelnuts, pecans, cashews)
- Peanut butter

Saturated fats are found in foods such as:
- High-fat cuts of meat (beef, lamb, pork)
- Chicken with the skin
- Whole-fat dairy products (milk and cream)
- Butter

- Cheese
- Ice cream
- Palm and coconut oil
- Lard

Trans-fats are found in foods such as:
- Commercially-baked pastries, cookies, doughnuts, muffins, cakes, pizza dough
- Packaged snack foods (crackers, microwave popcorn, chips)
- Stick margarine
- Vegetable shortening
- Fried foods (French fries, fried chicken, chicken nuggets, breaded fish)
- Candy bars

If you want to take up a healthy eating plan, trans-fat must be eradicated from your diet. Trans-fat can be found in a lot of junk and processed food, you can usually check by looking at the label on the product. You should also try to cut down on saturated fats which are found in full-fat dairy products and red meat, a great alternative is to have fish and poultry.

The amount of fat needed varies from person to person, based on what your lifestyle is like, your age, weight and how healthy you are. The USDA has a recommendation that you can use as a basic guideline:

- Limit the amount of trans-fat in your diet to 1% of your calorie intake – 2grams per day for a 2,000 calorie diet.
- Limit the amount of saturated fats you eat to less than 10% of your calories intake – 200 calories for a 2,000 calorie diet.
- Keep the intake of fat in your diet to 20-35% of calories.

Chapter 8: What Foods and Ingredients Should You Limit from Your Diet?

White Flour

White flour does not offer any nutritional value as it is highly processed and refined. Unlike other types of flour, white flour has been stripped of nutrition and the parts of the wheat kernel that aid digestion has been removed. This is also why your body processes it into blood sugar. The type of flours you should choose are ones that are not as processed, this way you can ensure that the grains are untouched. This includes foods like beans, lentils and wheat berries.

The process of making flour has changed significantly since the 19th century. Before that, flour was commonly made via a process of turning the grains by grinding it in between stones, and occasionally by a water wheel. The process was extremely time-consuming, with only the very rich being able to afford small amounts. As technology developed, machinery took over and high-steel high-speed rollers were used as they sped up the process while lowering the cost. This new method of processing is why white flour today is bad for our blood-sugar levels.

This modern way of processing food also turns grains into other highly processed foods including puffed corn snacks and cornflakes. Therefore, these types of processed foods will have a higher Glycemic Load (GL) than other less processed foods that have intact grains, popcorn being a great example, and other foods milled in a conventional way like whole-wheat flours.

Artificial Sweeteners and Refined Sugar

As part of a healthy eating plan, dieters are often told to limit their intake of sugar as a way to reduce calorie intake, maintain their weight and improve their health. This is why a lot of people find themselves turning to sugar substitutes and why there are so many types of artificial sweeteners on the market including: corn syrup, corn sweeteners, fructose, dextrose, invert sugar, maple syrup, molasses and maltose. Although artificial sweeteners tend to be synthetic, some are made from natural sources, however they tend to be a lot sweet than regular sugar.

Various beverages and food products also contain these products and are often labeled as "diet" or "sugar-free," including chewing gum, soft drinks, jellies, candy, fruit juice, yogurts and ice creams. As an alternative to sugar, they do have a few healthy benefits such as supporting weight loss and helping diabetes, as they tend to be really low in calories. However, more often than not, they actually increase your craving for sugar and can potentially have a negative effect on your health. Due to their popularity, a lot of research has gone into artificial sweeteners and their impact on health, and findings include possible links to certain types of cancer. Although, sweeteners may seem like a great alternative, it is better to limit them as much as possible and even think about eliminating your sugar intake all together.

Salt (Sodium Chloride)
Salt is a common ingredient found in most of the food we eat. If used consumed in little amounts, it can be good for your health as it is a source of iodine and sodium. Generally, one tablespoon of salt daily is sufficient, any more and it can potentially bad for your health. Therefore, monitoring the level of salt in your food is extremely important; you can do this by limiting the amount of salt in cooking and precooked food.

Foods that are high in salt tend to be highly processed, preserved in salt or salt-pickled and should be restricted from your healthy eating plan, or not eaten at all. As food labels tend to provide you with sodium levels instead of salt, you should note that 6 g of salt is equivalent to around 2400 mg of sodium. High blood pressure often occurs when more than 6 g of salt is consumed daily, eating 4.5g will reduce this risk, although 6 g per day is a great start. There is also sufficient evidence that suggests eating too much salt-pickled or food that has been preserved in salt increases the chance of developing stomach cancer.

Monosodium Glutamate (MSG)

MSG is a form of salt that has been chemically transformed into a flavor enhancer. A lot of studies have been carried out about the effects of MSG; with a significant finding linking it to processed foods and weight gain. MSG has this effect because it interferes with the hypothalamus - the part of the brain that regulates appetite – causing resistance to leptin, a hormone that controls appetite. When foods that contain MSG are consumed, the sense of being full up is lost, which leads to the craving of more food.

MSG is essentially an excitoxin, a chemical that causes over-stimulation in the brain, creating an excessive amount of dopamine. Dopamine is responsible for that drug-like rush associated with junk food, as it offers a quick sensation of happiness and is extremely addictive. This process is what causes addiction to junk food and overeating.

Cholesterol

High cholesterol is responsible for various health problems and can be found in foods that are high in fat as these have a high amount of cholesterol in them. Eating food that is high in cholesterol and saturated fat leads to cholesterol in the blood stream, which creates an accumulation of fatty plague on blood vessel walls. The presence of fatty plaque is what causes arteries to narrow, lose elasticity and ultimately become obstructed triggering a heart attack or stroke. By limiting the level of saturated fat in your diet, you will lower the risk of certain types of cancers including prostate and colon, and potentially breast cancer.

The major culprits of saturated fats in your diet are meat and dairy products and certain types of oil – palm, palm kernel and coconut – also contain a high amount of saturated fats unlike vegetable oils. You can reduce your intake by eating healthier alternatives to these food products like swapping red meat for poultry and fish, and whole-fat dairy products for a low-fat alternative. Increasing your intake of fruit, vegetables and cereals into your diet is also useful.

Processed Food

Over 60% of adults can be classed as overweight or obese, with the main culprit being the amount of readily available processed foods including favorites like fries, hamburgers, pizza, cookies, ice cream and potato chips. Eating a lot of process foods put you at risk of becoming obese and developing related illnesses such as heart disease, high blood pressure and diabetes. It may not seem like a lot of food, but eating a hamburger and fries, washed down with your favorite soft drink is laden with sugar, trans-fat, salt and is also calorific. It may surprise you but an average-sized 12-ounce soft drink is filled with over 30 grams of sugar, with the recommended daily intake being only 20 grams. Although, our body converts sugar into energy, these types of foods and beverages eating in high amounts are extremely bad for your health.

A lot of processed foods contain a high amount of hydrogenated and trans-fat which are used to extend their shelf life, but unfortunately, this also raises your cholesterol, clogs your arteries and increases your risk of heart disease. Processed food designed for children – pasta mixes, chicken noodle soup, alphabet soup and so on- is particularly bad as they tend to contain a high amount of MSG.

Frozen Foods & Canned Goods

Limiting the amount of frozen foods in your diet is important as they are not as healthy and wholesome as fresh foods. This is because frozen foods tend to be processed, with additives and artificial ingredients. Additionally, they generally contain a high level of salt, which can increase your risk of developing hypertension or a stroke. It has also been said that during the freezing process, food loses its nutritional value.

Canned foods are often made to last a long time, which is evident by their expiry date, indicating that they are highly processed. What makes these foods last for so long is the preservatives that are added to them, salt and sugar being a key ingredient. This process also reduces the amount of nutrients in canned food, particularly potassium and vitamin C.

Margarine & Hydrogenated Oils

Margarine, often used as an alternative to butter, is highly artificial. Although it has always been used as a healthier substitute, research has no shown that it is not as healthy as you think. Health conditions like heart disease are becoming increasingly wide spread and are often as a result of consuming too much hydrogenated food and margarine – foods that have been made with an extended shelf life. This also includes products such as cookies, crackers, baked goods, frozen meals etc.

Margarine is made by hydrogenation, a process that pushes hydrogen atoms through holes of unsaturated fat. The hydrogen gas is pressurized, then bubbled via vegetable oil, with the support of a metal catalyst, often platinum, nickel or sometimes another type of metal. Once the hydrogen atoms are mixed with the carbon atom, the vegetable oil hardens or saturates. This process creates a new product, margarine, which is grey and smells rotten. The metals used in this process are highly toxic, and regardless of how careful the process is carried out, a small amount of it will always be retained in the margarine. Often, to mask the smell and disguise the grey coloring, a deodorant and dye is used.

As well this, hydrogenated oils and even ones that have only been partially hydrogenated can be linked to cancer, diabetes and heart conditions. They hinder the absorption of essential fatty acids, a vital chemical needed in the body for it to function efficiently.

Caffeinated Products

While drinking coffee, tea and other carbonated products may seem harmless; they can be quite addictive because they contain a high content of caffeine. Your average cup of coffee will contain nearly 100mg of caffeine, although this can vary between 40 and 170mg. Your average cup of tea will contain 27mg, but again can vary between 8 and 91mg.

In essence, caffeine is like a drug and shares similarities with other addictive products, like nicotine, alcohol and other drugs, pharmacologically affecting us in the same way. But, unlike those other products, coffee is not frowned upon and is an integral part of our daily lives. Therefore, we are unlikely to question the impact it has on our health.

As well as being addictive, studies also show that even a small amount of coffee can wreak a significant amount of havoc on our health. It can cause sperm damage, reducing the chances of fertility. It is also dangerous to drink while you are pregnant as it affects the amount of rest the baby receives, potentially leading to behavioral problems later in life. In small doses, caffeine can lower the heart rate, but in a large concentration can actually cause the heart to beat at an abnormally fast rate. It is also a powerful diuretic, making you urinate more often, which is down to the increase of blood flow in the kidneys. If you are having troubles with sleeping, caffeine will make it worse as it causes insomnia.

Artificial Additives, Dyes & Preservatives
The choice of substances added to our food is increasingly gaining attention due to the growing concern about the safety of the chemicals used. Consumers are constantly being exposed to an unregulated combination of artificial additives, dyes and preservatives on a regular basis. With most people buying commercially packaged products that contain a mixture of chemicals that are unregulated, they are unaware of the health risks posed.

Although each chemical has been tested separately to see how it reacts with humans, as a cocktail of chemicals they have not been thoroughly tested. What this means is that while one of the chemicals are safe for human consumption, combined with other chemicals there is no clear definition of what impact they potentially have. In 2000, some research was carried out that examined the mixture of four food additives, and a combination of six artificial food colors, with toxic found in both.

Cheese
Cheese is a major source of saturated fat and can be found in most foods, from sandwiches to healthy salads. It is actually said to be more harmful than beef or butter. People eat cheese believing that its calcium-richness has plenty of health benefits, but in reality, they would be much better of getting their calcium intake from low –fat products or fortified orange juice.

Although, it can seem like a struggle to avoid cheese, it is best to reduce your intake. You can do this by not adding it to your food and ordering food from restaurants without the cheese. Even when you order a pizza, you can ask them to put half the amount of cheese on it, and stuffed-crust should be avoided at all costs.

Soda & Other Carbonated Drinks

Carbonated beverages are produced through the injection of carbon dioxide into water under pressure. Essentially, carbon dioxide is a waste product and is known to kill healthy cells. As well as carbonated drinks containing carbon dioxide, they also do not offer any nutrients, but instead are packed full of refined sugar, which can potentially damage your kidneys. It has also been suggested that these drinks weaken your immune system, and the caffeine in them is addictive which increases your heart rate and damages the nervous system.

Carbonated drinks also contain phosphoric acid, which is bad for your teeth and bones because it depletes calcium. As these drinks are typically processed, they contain preservatives and artificial chemicals used to flavor. These can also cause health problems from simple allergies to obesity, diabetes, tooth decay, osteoporosis and even cancer.

Alcohol & Cigarettes

Drinking alcohol and/or smoking poses a variety of health risks including problems with the liver, upper aero-digestive tract and cancer. They increase the risk of developing cancers of the oral cavity and throat, using them together increases the risk. This is because the mouth and throat are areas in your body that smoke and drink are exposed to.

Alcohol can damage your liver, but also increases the potential risk of DNA damage, this in turn causes cells to mutate and uncontrollably multiply which can not only cause cancer to develop, but has also been linked to stroke. Chronic drinkers also face damaging their nervous system, which can lead to dementia. Pregnant women should limit their intake of alcohol, or eliminate completely, as heavy drinking can cause Fetal Alcohol Syndrome, considered to be the cause of several physical defects and behavioral conditions.

Chapter 9: Choosing Food That Is Nutritionally Good For You

Fruit and Vegetables
Fruit and vegetables are great for your health as they are packed full of nutrients that will keep you healthy, by boosting your immune system and supporting digestion.

Antibiotic & Hormone Free Meat
Animals are seen as a commodity and treated the same way. They are pumped with antibiotics, covered in pesticides and fed growth hormones to speed up the production process and enhance their productiveness. These chemicals once in the animal are eventually transferred to us when we eat meat, which can be extremely bad for our health. Instead of eating this type of meat, there is meat readily available from animals that have been bred through cleaner farming under humane conditions. This is meat is much better for you.

Unprocessed Food
Unprocessed foods are foods that are natural and have not been tampered with, these include raw or steam vegetables, fresh fruit, lean meat, poultry and whole grains.

Use Butter Rather Than Margarine

Although butter is seen as an unhealthy food, eating it in small portions it is completely healthy. Butter is less processed than margarine and so does not post as many health risks. It is also rich in trace minerals like selenium, an antioxidant. Butter also contains iodine, vitamin A and fatty acids.

Olive Oil

Olive oil is extremely good for your health and offers so many nutritional benefits. It does wonders for strengthening the immune system, protecting your body from viruses and various diseases. Olive oil also contains phytonutrient, which is a chemical that imitates the effect of ibuprofen in the reduction of inflammation.

Beans

Beans are packed full of protein, fiber and water, leaving you feeling fuller faster which means adding them to your meal will help you reduce your calorie intake. Beans also have low sugar content, which prevent your insulin from spiking stopping hunger pangs.

Seeds & Nuts

Seeds and nuts are full of nutrients and you only really need a handful for perfect dose of fats, vitamins and minerals, which all contribute to a healthy heart, brain and waistline. Seeds and nuts are also full of fiber, which supports digestion and leaves you feeling fuller for longer. Ensure that you eat unprocessed forms of nuts, i.e. without added sugar or salt.

Yogurt

Yogurt may be made from milk, but it has a whole lot more nutrients. It is rich in calcium, protein, riboflavin, vitamin B12 and vitamin B6. The live cultures found in yoghurt are great at preventing antibiotic-related diarrhea. Eating yogurt is great for all ages; it offers children a balanced source of carbohydrates, fat, protein and minerals. For older people, who may suffer from a sensitive colon it is also a beneficial food to eat.

Whole Grain

Whole grain products have always been considered to be healthy. They contain a small amount of saturated fats and so are good for heart health. They also reduce the risk of developing certain cancers, particularly colon and stomach cancer. Whole grain is good for people that suffer from diabetes as it regulates the bowels and supports the intestinal function.

Fish

Omega-3 fatty acids occur naturally in the majority of fish, making fish great for your health. Fish also contains a high level of amino acids, protein and bioactive peptides, calcitonin which aids in the regulation and stabilization of minerals and collagen in the bone and the tissue around it. It is also suggested that people who regularly eat fish reduce their risk of developing certain types of cancers.

White & Green Teas

The Chinese have been drinking white and green tea for centuries because they are aware of all the health benefits that they have. They are packed with anti-oxidants which can help reduce the risk of developing lung, skin and colon cancer. They also work great against the effects of smoking, through reversing cellular damage. White and green tea also decrease skin damage, which is why a lot of skin care products have green and white tea as part of their ingredients. Drinking at least three to four cups of green tea a day could help you burn an extra 70 calories, around 500 additional calories a week.

Natural Juices

Natural fruit and vegetable juices are rich in nutrients including vitamin C, potassium and folate. Natural juices that have been fortified with calcium are even better, especially for those that suffer with intolerance to lactose; some are even rich in vitamin D, which supports the absorption of calcium in the body. Drinking natural juices is also a great way for you to get your daily portion of fruit and vegetables without having to eat them.

Water with a Lemon Twist

Drinking water is an essential part of a healthy eating plan, but if you are fed up with its tastelessness, try adding a lemon slice. Not only will this make it tastier, lemon also enhances the detoxifying effect, cleansing the body of toxic impurities while preventing the breakdown of tissue and growth of bacteria. It is also good for those that suffer from inflammation in the joints, as it helps to dissolve uric acid and other toxins, malaria gout, tuberculosis and rickets.

Lemon is good for the liver as it helps with stimulation, but also, when the liver enzymes are too diluted it provides a natural strengthening agent. It also regulates the level of oxygen and calcium in the liver, which essentially helps the blood.

Adding lemon to water also aids the digestion process as lemon can ease symptoms of indigestion like wind, bloating and heartburn. It also supports the elimination of waste from the bowels in a more efficient way, therefore, alleviating or preventing diarrhea, constipation and a whole load of other gastrointestinal conditions.

As well as the benefits mentioned above, lemon water also helps to:

- Purify blood.
- Lower blood pressure.
- Reduce phlegm.
- Ease symptoms of allergies, asthma and other respiratory-related conditions.
- Dissolve kidney stones, gallstones, calcium deposits and pancreatic stones.

Chapter 10: Healthy Options When Eating Out

The majority of us enjoy eating out, but the food that we choose to buy when we do is often laden with fat, salt, cholesterol and sugar. As part of a healthy eating plan, you should be cautious when you go to a restaurant, only choosing healthy options, or asking for special request when ordering – this may be you asking for dressing or sauces to be placed on the side, rather than over your meal. This way you have the option of whether you eat it or not.

When ordering from a menu, choose dishes that have been prepared in a healthy way whether that is steamed, roasted, poached, baked, grilled or broiled as they are likely to have less fat in them. As tempting as it may be, you should avoid foods that are creamy, buttered, fried or marinated in oil, as they will be dishes that are laden with fat and the wrong type of nutrients. You do not have to feel like you are restricting yourself but can instead make wise choices, for example, rather than ordering a fried egg with French toast, you can have a poached egg with whole wheat toast and jam.

Due to the growing number of health conscious diners, restaurants are beginning to put a healthy selection of dishes on their menus, special salads being a favorite. Although salads have long been seen as a side dish, there are salads that act as main meals and may come with other food such as cottage cheese, pasta salad, guacamole, diced ham, hard cheese and olives. Ensure that you only eat a small amount of foods as these can undo the healthiness of the salad. As salad often comes with dressing, try to stick with a low-calorie alternative, you could even skin the dressing and sprinkle some pepper or add a hint of lemon.

While restaurants offer healthy alternatives on their menu, fast food restaurants tend not to. Although, there may be an option that seems like a healthy, more often than not, it is still high in fat, salt, sugar and other processed goods.

Chapter 11: What Exercises Should You Do?

Everyone needs to incorporate physical activity into their lives if they want to improve and maintain their health. Exercising regularly helps cut the risk of developing diseases, while strengthening the bones and increasing the metabolism. It is especially good as a way of releasing stress. There are many types of exercises you can do and the great thing about exercise is that you can start of slow and gradually increase your work out, and then you will find that you actually reach the stage of enjoying it.

Running/Walking/Hiking

The best thing about running is that it is inexpensive – you will have to buy a suitable pair of running shoes – and it is an excellent form of physical exercise. Running is extremely good for the cardiovascular system; it supports bone health and also is good for maintaining and losing weight. If you have never ran before, or not for a long time, you will need to start of slow. Begin by going for a brisk walk, and then slowly build it up by jogging and then eventually running. It will take a long time, but you need to stick with it all the way.

To make it easier and more enjoyable, you could ask a friend to run with you, you could also sign up to your local running club, this makes sure that you commit. Most clubs have events that you can compete in, to bring out your competitive nature. They will also have a session that is specifically designed for those who are just starting out; they also cater to all age groups and abilities. If you want to mix it up a bit, you could join an orienteering club instead, this way you get to combine runn ng with navigating in different environments.

Cycling

Riding a bike is a really good work out, but also a great method of transport. Providing that where you live is safe to ride a bike, you could cycle to visit friends or family; you could even commute to work. Although you could also cycle in the gym, or for leisure, cycling when you have to go somewhere is great because if you are a busy person, it saves you a lot of time but you also get your work out. It will also save you money, by saving on petrol or public transport.

Swimming

Swimming is one of the best exercises there are for various reasons. Water is good for the body and is seen as a relaxing medium, it eases aches and pains and creates a sense of calmness. As a form of exercise, it works in the same way as resistance training as your body has to work against the water. It is considered to be one of the superior forms of exercises in relation to burning extra calories, toning muscles and general fitness.

Unlike riding a bike, swimming can be learnt regardless of your age. If you are thinking of picking up swimming, but don't know how to swim, consider going to a few classes or hiring a swimming instructor to help you learn some techniques. Once you become comfortable and confident in the water, you will find yourself learning how to control your body and how to hold your breath. It is extremely beneficial as knowing how to swim is an essential skill.

To start out, you may want to practice swimming in shallow water until you are comfortable with moving your muscles while submerged in water. You can then move on to the deeper end of the pool. Remember, you should never go into a pool after a meal, and especially after drinking alcohol. Also, never swim in cold water or open waters such as lakes or the ocean.

Competitive & Team Sports

Participating in a team sport is not only great fun, but it will also teach you valuable life skills like accountability, leadership, dedication and most importantly team effort. It will also bring out your competitive nature that will make yourself push even harder, making your exercise session a lot more effective. There are various team sports that you can participate in from soccer to baseball, if you are unsure of where to start you should consider join a local club, that way you can develop and practice with a team. Participating in team sports is good for your health and can also help boost your self-esteem as you work hard and achieve goals.

Going to the Gym

Joining a gym is good for those of you that dislike the outdoors, but not ideal for those of you who find it difficult to get into a routine and stick to it. Once you join a gym, you have to ensure that go it is all about commitment.

When you go to the gym, you will need to get an induction to learn how to use the machines, especially if you have never stepped foot inside a gym before. Once you know how to use the equipment, begin with a five to ten minute warm up, so your body adjusts to the workout. You do not need to over exert yourself as doing a set of ten or twenty is just fine. You will probably find yourself getting bored of the same routine so mixing it up a bit each session, or each week will make sure that you never find boring, otherwise you will be put off of going.

When you are just starting out, limit yourself to five to 10 machines, spending around fifteen to twenty minutes on each. Try not to take a break between machines, as you do not want your heart rate to decrease too much. Stick with machines as opposed to free weights, particularly if you are a beginner as you could end up hurting yourself. Lifting weights should only really be for the experienced user.

Summary

With so much information available about health and nutrition, it is becoming increasingly difficult to keep track. The aim of this book was to present the basics of nutrition as a guideline for you to take away and keep in mind. Ensuring that you live a healthy lifestyle along with a balanced diet will reduce the risks of developing various diet-related illnesses, while making sure that you remain in optimum health, physically and mentally. Hopefully, add years to your life.

It is a common misconception that only people who suffer from chronic health conditions need to worry about what they eat and the nutrition in their diet, but that is simply not true. Following a healthy eating plan can benefit everyone and is a way of preventing any chronic conditions from developing. This includes all age groups, as children's diets should also be closely monitored to ensure that they are nutritionally balanced, otherwise they may suffer from weight-related issues too. They should be eating food that supplies them with carbohydrates, proteins, vitamins, minerals and other key nutrients. Likewise, an elderly person should have a diet that has a sufficient amount of nutrients and anti-oxidants that can fight against the inevitable process of ageing. It will also increase their mobility, which in turn leads to a better life. Pregnant woman also need to follow a healthy eating plan to safeguard the health of her and her baby, insufficient nutrients can lead to various health problems including birth abnormalities in the baby, and deficiencies for the mother including calcium and iron.

The various physical activities mentioned in this book are also aimed at all ages and abilities. Participating in regular exercise is an essential part of a healthy lifestyle, as it will enhance the effects of your diet. People who live a sedentary life are unlikely to live as long as those who regularly exercise, as idleness can lead to the development of coronary heart disease and a whole list of other health problems. It has even been said that not doing any physical activity puts you in nearly as much danger as smoking when it comes to heart disease, hypertension and cholesterol. As well as enhancing your physical appearances and keeping you healthy, it is also a great way to distress. Exercise releases endorphins, which will leave you feeling really good.

Hopefully, having read this book, you are ready to change your relationship with food and exercise for the better. Remember, it will be hard to begin with, but you need to stick with it and be consistent; you will soon start to see and feel the benefits of living a healthy life. All you have to do is take the next step.

www.ingramcontent.com/pod-product-compliance
Lightning Source LLC
Chambersburg PA
CBHW071004290526
45795CB00005B/1768